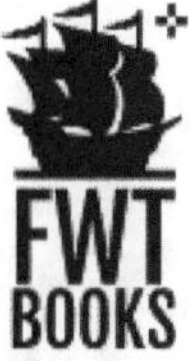

FWT BOOKS

Published in November, 2019

by Lorna B. Stuart, M.D.

Designed

by Flat World Technology Philadelphia

In the small town of Phoenixville in the suburbs of Philadelphia, you will find a nonprofit medical clinic founded to serve those in the community without health insurance. Aptly and simply named The Clinic, it has been providing free medical care to thousands of patients every year since opening its doors in 2002.

The Clinic has only a handful of paid staff, but over 120 volunteers – doctors, nurses, clerical and more. These devoted individuals provide, on average, 8,000 patient visits each year. These devoted individuals change lives.

The Clinic was founded to be, and remains to this day, a place of compassion and caring. It acts as a safety net for the most vulnerable in the Phoenixville community. Our doctors and nurses see patients walk through the front door sick, defeated and frightened. Some have not seen a doctor in years or decades. Some have never been to a doctor in their lives. These patients all leave The Clinic with not only the promise of health, but hope as well.

Around 28 million people in the United States lack health insurance. These individuals include part-time workers who cannot get full-time hours (and benefits), new citizens, college graduates still looking for decent jobs, contractors who are in business for themselves and many others who simply cannot afford health insurance. With some health insurance premiums rivalling the cost of a mortgage, people choose to go without benefits and therefore without medical care. Without access to medical care, preventative care doesn't happen, minor problems are not treated until they become major issues, a job must be declined because it requires a physical exam and an appendix may rupture, turning a simple operation into a several-day hospitalization.

The Clinic's founders believe that everyone deserves a kind, competent home for his or her health care. Until these services are accessible to all, The Clinic will be there to provide compassionate care.

The Founding of The Clinic

Early in my medical career, I remember watching the movie Patch Adams, engrossed by the story of the title character's establishment of a clinic in West Virginia, free of restrictions. No insurance forms. No malpractice. Nothing but medical care the way it should be.

"Wow!" I thought, "that would be so great. I want to do that."

In 1980, I had established a solo medical practice in a

blue-collar town about 30 miles west of Philadelphia. During the first years of my practice, billing was very straightforward: there were no HMOs in the area, insurance was primarily for hospitalization and office fees were inexpensive enough that most people were able to pay by cash or check. There was always freedom to accommodate an indigent patient or two. Twenty years into medical practice, I was becoming more and more dissatisfied with how I had to run my office. Formularies, insurance restrictions and refusals to pay for services, patients buffeted from one plan to another with any change in employment and cranky administrators with no medical education telling physicians what tests could be ordered were just a few of the aggravations to be faced on a daily basis.

By 2000, the town had grown and my practice had as well, now with three doctors and a nurse practitioner. An Ivy League Hospital had purchased it in 1995, and fees had been raised without our input, multiple HMOs had been incorporated and despite promises to the contrary, we had begun to be micromanaged.

Insurance companies might come in, unannounced, expect to see a dozen randomly-chosen charts of "their" patients, then leave a report of perceived deficits to our excellent and legible charting. One final straw came when an insurance company subordinate denied paying us for a vaccine we had given because the nurse had not recorded the time she had given it to the patient. Date, nurse's signature and doctor's signature were insufficient – no time recorded meant a refusal to pay.

As these indignities ever increased, I was also seeing more and more patients who were putting off medical care, even for their children. They were sometimes forced to choose whether to see a doctor or to buy their family's groceries for the week. With the acquisition of our practice by the Ivy League, we were no longer permitted to see patients without charge.

My outrage was nearly complete when I saw a sick seven-year-old child on a Friday afternoon, a lovely little girl who was feverish and dehydrated and sick enough with tonsillitis to have missed a whole week of school. As I gently suggested to the parents that next time they might bring her in earlier, their embarrassment was acute when they said they hoped she would get better on her own, as they did not know how to both pay for a doctor visit and get their groceries.

At that time, there were about 45 million people in the United States who did not have health insurance. All over, there were parents agonizing over taking a sick child to the doctor. All over, there were people unable to treat their diabetes, hypertension, or pneumonia without running up serious debt.

Enough was enough.

In this same town, once bustling in the 19th century steel industry, there was a large Episcopal Church and adjacent three-story Victorian mansion of a rectory, suitable for a rector's family and his half dozen children. St. Peter's Church was still active, but the rectory had been abandoned – too large, too expensive to heat in the winter and impossible to cool in the summer. The large windows had been boarded up, the furnace no longer worked and the water had been turned off. The roof was so damaged that water dripped into the third floor, through the ceiling of the second floor and plants and weeds were growing tall in one of the second floor bedrooms. Local children were frightened to walk by this boarded-up eyesore, scared that it might be a haunted house. Since safe demolition of this once lovely building would have a price tag of $75,000, the church could not even afford to have it torn down.

In 1998, a new rector was appointed, and for the first

time in St. Peter's history, that new rector was a woman. When Reverend Marie Swayze and I first met the following year, we bonded over our perceived need for real social change in the community. We started a food pantry in the church and she would occasionally bring an indigent patient to see me in my office on a Sunday afternoon.

We knew more was needed. We knew much more was needed.

One day, we sat together on a low stone wall between the church and the rectory while I bemoaned my dissatisfaction with the economics of modern medicine. Inspiration struck and I blurted out, "Let's start a clinic!"

"OK, let's do it!" came her enthusiastic reply.

The Reverend Swayze knew how to tackle the legal hoops, and I was able to make comprehensive lists of medical equipment and people we would require. The location was a no-brainer, as the new rector had been agonizing over the misuse of the historic rectory.

An optimistic estimate for creating a clinic out of the shell of this building was about $200,000. We met with an entrepreneur whose daughter I had helped years earlier, a man who asked to remain anonymous. About 30 seconds into our elevator pitch, he stopped us. "I'll give you $100,000 now and another $100,000 next quarter." Those were the magic words. We got to work immediately, stabilizing the roof and obtaining contractor estimates.

In the end, it would cost nearly twice the original optimistic sum and take twice as long as expected to turn our dreams for the building into a reality. We raised funds in any way we could – we sent out mailers, talked to churches and service clubs and held jumble sales and spaghetti dinners. I agreed to work at no salary at all for the first months. Finally, a woman who had lived in the rectory as a child contacted us and gave an enormously generous gift so that her once-beloved home would thrive again as The Clinic.

We certainly had detractors. Many major foundations would not provide funding for at least two years after opening, out of concern that we might not be successful.

Nevertheless, we were. The spaghetti dinner hosted by a veteran's group netted $350. An elderly woman sent a card and a crumpled $5 bill. A book sale brought us $500. Pharmaceutical companies gave drug samples and donated equipment. We received small donations and large gifts alike, along with a huge outpouring of support from our community. In October of 2002, we proudly and lovingly opened our doors to care for anyone without medical insurance.

As we became more established and our reputation

grew, corporate donors came on board, and foundations began to show interest in our work. Other churches regularly sent gifts and volunteers, and individual donors in our community became our lifeblood for daily operational funds.

One of our earliest volunteer doctors, internist Dr. Susan Prouty, became a valued salaried physician as soon as we could afford to pay another staff member. A former pharmaceutical rep named Mary Ellen Smith became a volunteer on the second day we were open and became Lab Manager, organizing and supervising our lab and pharmacy. She was also instrumental is obtaining some major publicity for The Clinic, including CNN, NBC interviews and a spot in People Magazine. Artist and friend Anne Reid designed and decorated The Clinic to establish a warm and inviting place and then continued on as Volunteer Coordinator for many years. Eventually, we were able to hire full-time nurses and administrative staff as well, though volunteers remain the strong core of our staff.

From the beginning and still to this day, we follow one precept: If you do not have insurance, you are welcome. No screening for income. No established fees. No screening social security numbers. Patients are asked to donate only what they can afford – for some patients that is nothing, and that's ok.   A large world map on our wall allows patients to place a pin where they have come from, and more than 70 countries are now highlighted!

The Clinic provides compassionate care, regardless of the circumstances that have brought our patients to us. This, in my opinion, is exactly how to be a doctor!

Chapter One: Heart Attack

She puffed her way up the four steps to the front door, pulling herself up with the handrail. The Clinic was not open yet, but through the glass-paned door, we saw her coming, struggling. As we let her in, she gasped, "Help me. I can't breathe. I just have bronchitis, I know it. I just need some antibiotics so I can go to work."

The woman was an overweight diabetic in her mid-forties who held down three part-time jobs, including her favorite, a corner crossing guard for elementary school children.

Rushing her into the closest exam room, we grabbed the oxygen and EKG machine and hooked her up. We got an aspirin into her while we read the tracing. This was no case of bronchitis – the woman was having a heart attack in our Clinic!

After calling for an ambulance, we continued to monitor her blood pressure and oxygen levels. An examination of her lungs revealed rales, the crackling sound due to moisture in the lungs from congestive heart failure. She was in deep trouble.

But when the ambulance crew arrived, she started to panic.

"No, I won't go to the hospital! I can't go to the hospital! I don't have any insurance. I can't pay them. I already owe them money!" she cried.

She was adamant and continued to refuse the ambulance until the arrival of her 18-year-old son. "Mom, I want you to live. I want you to see me graduate next month," he pleaded. Grudgingly, she allowed the ambulance staff to put her onto the gurney and take her to the hospital.

She stayed about three days in the local hospital and had two stents placed in her coronary arteries. Within a week, she was back at her corner as a crossing guard. How many things are wrong with this picture? She was terrified at the thought of having to go to a hospital since she could not pay. She could have been at the hospital an hour earlier or maybe more if she had gone straight from her home. She probably would have had less heart muscle damage without that delay in treatment. She had felt excluded from a hospital system meant to serve her when she was very ill.

She had three part-time jobs – one actually in the cafeteria of that local hospital where she received care! However, none of those three jobs offered health insurance benefits. She had applied and asked again and again for more hours, but despite her excellent work ethic, she was never given enough hours to allow her access to a medical benefit plan.

This woman – a hard-working, tax-paying citizen – was denied the most basic, lifesaving health care, and our current health care system had made her feel helpless. Despite doing everything right, the system had failed her completely.

The risk factors of heart disease have been very clearly delineated. Hypertension, diabetes, lack of exercise, obesity, high cholesterol and smoking are well-known contributing factors. It is far less expensive to treat these risk factors with regular, affordable primary care than to pay for a single Cardiac Intensive Care Unit admission.

The cost of many blood pressure medications is very small: chain pharmacies have standard medications for around $10 for a three-month supply. Similarly, some of the generic medications for cholesterol and diabetes are covered for around the same price. Compare that to an ambulance ride ($400+), an emergency evaluation

($800-$2,000), radiology, stress tests, CCU days (at $3,000-5,000 a day) and more costs associated with emergency care. The price of a few preventative offices visits, lab tests and medications is significantly cheaper for the hospital and the state, and clearly better for the wellbeing of patients.

Chapter Two: Diabetic Emergency

One day, a local landscaping contractor sent one of his employees to The Clinic when he was clipping rhododendron bushes and became confused. Oddly, he did not seem to know how to use the clipping shears anymore. The man had always been a good worker, and this behavior was out of the ordinary.

The staff and volunteers at The Clinic knew immediately that this man was truly ill, even though he spoke only a little English.

As we took his vital signs, we noted that his pulse was quite rapid and that he was sweating all over. He did not have a fever but his tongue was dry. A three-second blood sugar result gave us the answer: his blood sugar was more than six times the normal value! His vision was so blurry from the elevated glucose that it was little wonder that he could not see to use his shears properly. This man would be dead in another week or two without urgent help.

In a private medical practice, one might send him to the local hospital emergency department for intravenous hydration, an insulin drip to bring his sugar level down slowly and continual monitoring of his electrolytes: sodium, potassium and magnesium. He might have been admitted for a few days to adjust insulin levels, while having cardiac monitoring and a host of other endocrine blood tests. He might have an abdominal scan to examine his pancreas.

But he didn't have any medical insurance.

He worked for $14 an hour, some 50 hours a week, and that was just enough to rent a room for himself and his wife and buy groceries and some basic necessities. How could be buy medical insurance? He could not even afford car insurance.

We treated this critically ill man as an outpatient, starting with an intravenous infusion of saline since he was so severely dehydrated. Multiple small doses of fast-acting insulin were given and we monitored his blood sugars as they slowly came down over the next few hours. His cardiogram remained normal, despite expected abnormal potassium and sodium levels. We were able to send off blood samples but knew that we would not obtain an answer about his magnesium level or kidney function until the next day.

As his sugar dipped into the 300s and he was feeling physically much better, we gave him exact instructions as to what to eat for the next two meals. He was also given a blood-glucose monitoring kit and a supply of short-acting insulin to use. We saw him first thing next morning, and his sugar was now in the 200s. Much safer! We all breathed a sigh of relief.

Why did this happen? If he had had some basic health coverage, a doctor could have seen him when he first began feeling ill. Instead, he tried to ignore the symptoms. Had he become comatose and taken to a hospital by ambulance, he would have had tens of thousands of dollars of tests, CT scans and an ICU stay. His bill for an inpatient stay would have exceeded $100,000, an amount he could never have paid off. The burden of that debt would have had a damaging effect on his life, his family and his health.

Instead, good fortune shone on him the day he found us at The Clinic, and he was treated by compassionate doctors and nurses without concern for his ability to pay.

Chapter 3: Bipolar Depression

There are few disorders as misunderstood as bipolar disorder. Most psychiatric experts feel that this illness is related to imbalance in the neurotransmitters, the chemicals of the brain. Disparities of serotonin, dopamine and norepinephrine cause a variety of symptoms, such as easy anger, deep depression, rapidly changing mood and significant anxiety. Quite commonly, traumatic incidents in a person's life may trigger these hormonal imbalances, but genetics also play a role. Whatever the cause, the disorder comes at no fault of the patient.

Bipolar mood disorder might be quite severe or can be seen in a milder form. A primary care physician's awareness of the disorder and familiarity with its various treatments can mean a new life for those who suffer from it. At The Clinic, in treating patients without health insurance, we see a huge number of patients whose bipolar illness make access to a good job with job security (and accompanying medical benefits) nearly impossible.

Near The Clinic, there is a small college, and its students without medical insurance are frequently sent to us. The college's social worker sent one student, a young woman from Tennessee, to us. She clearly had symptoms of severe anxiety. She could not finish assignments, chewed her fingers and scratched her face to the point that it always had skin lesions. She initially told us she could not sleep, but as we got to know her and build her trust, she told us about a horrific childhood.

Abused sexually, physically and mentally, she was forced to go every day after school to a family friend's home where much of the abuse occurred. She hinted to her parents that this was not a good place, but the hints were ignored and the abuse continued.

Somehow, she was able to finish high school and, two or three years later, she found herself in Pennsylvania at this small Christian university. When she became a patient at The Clinic, we were able to diagnose her anxiety as a symptom of bipolar disorder, and once this was treated, she was able to finish college over a seven-year period. On the day of her graduation, two of The Clinic's staff were there to see her walk across the stage. If her bipolar illness had not been treated, it is possible that she would have wound up a welfare recipient, with a family that she, in turn, reflexively abused.

Anxiety and depression are two of the most common issues needing treatment at The Clinic. Depression, especially combined with anxiety, can cause people to spiral out of control and lose employment. Loss of a job often means loss of self-esteem, which in turn results in a loss of motivation and can lead to even longer unemployment.

There is still an enormous tendency to blame the patient for the depression. The patient hears:

"Just go out and do something."

"Everyone feels anxious – just get over it."

But it is the neurotransmitters in the brain that are dictating the mood disorder. Certainly, cognitive therapy and positive feedback are helpful, but the underlying physiologic condition must be treated as well.

Treating psychiatric disorders is still more of an art than a science. There are no lab tests, no chemical markers and no physical changes in the body. So many clinicians find this a daunting task. Trained to rely on lab tests and other quantitative assessments of conditions, the qualitative symptoms are more difficult to pin down for a diagnosis. However, very often, careful exploration of the symptoms will present the answer. Psychiatry is nearly out of reach for many Americans with insurance; for the uninsured, it is altogether impossible to access. Primary care doctors, more and more, must be at the forefront of diagnosis and treatment, and at The Clinic, we strive to provide this care in every instance we can.

Chapter Four: Trauma

A blistered and painful burn. A deep cut from a sharp knife. An ankle turned and sprained. What to do? Where to go?

When The Clinic was first opened in 2002, there were no urgent care centers in the area. The only options for an urgent injury were the emergency department of the local hospital or a doctor's office, if you were able to get in immediately.   Even after a few walk-in urgent care centers opened within a few miles of The Clinic, cost and transportation often made such a trip impossible for our patients.

The Clinic was in the center of a town with infrequent bus service. Many people had no car, or just one car in a household, which was used by someone else to go to work. Many of our patients walked to The Clinic to receive care.

During a routine day at The Clinic, I was always pleased to be able to sew up a laceration, treat a burn or other urgent medical issue and send the patient home with all of his or her necessary supplies. When the receptionist would send a message back that "someone is here and bleeding" or "a patient is here who can't walk," I was happy to know that they had found us and that we could help.

Too many people without insurance might choose to self-treat even a deep and bleeding cut, but the result is so often infection, which can lead to further tissue injury.

One diabetic patient at The Clinic worked as a laborer and had lost much of the feeling in his feet. He came in to see us with a deep, ulcerated area on the sole of his right foot. He had not felt it, but saw that his sock was sticking to his foot and used a mirror to find the ulcer. The ulcer was nearly to the bone and we knew that our chances of success were low, but started him on antibiotics, wound care and gave him bags of bandaging and new clean white socks. After a few weeks, his foot showed little progress, and in the end, he required an amputation of part of his foot. We continued with follow-up visits, providing him with medical care and the bandaging that he would not have been able to afford. This man was able to return to his job, instead of dying of sepsis.

Sprained ankles are also a common problem at The Clinic. Most times, a sprained ankle does not need an X-ray, just a careful examination. However, what about splints, elastic bandages and crutches? Barely-used crutches are frequently donated to The Clinic and these are a huge help, as we can show the person how to use the crutches correctly while he or she is still in the building. Generous donors also provide canes and walkers so that we are able to provide complete treatment in one visit.

Lack of medical insurance will frequently cause a

patient to put off treatment until the illness or injury reaches an advanced state. One day, a man came in limping, his left foot painful and swollen. A week earlier, he had stepped on a wood screw and it penetrated the sole of his shoe. He had gone to an urgent care clinic, but was provided with a prescription for antibiotics, not free samples. The prescription alone would cost $300! He certainly couldn't pay that, so he decided to go without. By the time we saw him, the entire front of his foot was badly infected: red, warm, tender and swollen. After we'd evaluated him, we were able to give him a powerful antibiotic and would see him back the next day. Thankfully, his foot was saved and hospitalization was prevented.

"An ounce of prevention is worth a pound of cure." Benjamin Franklin's adage is perfectly represented by the story of this patient and so many others that find themselves at The Clinic.

Chapter Five: Compassion For All Humans

One morning, a young woman who spoke little to no English arrived at our door. She was clearly in pain, her feet wrapped up in white bandaging. She limped and there were tears in the corners of her eyes. "Puede ayudarme?" (Can you help me?)

In response, we helped her into the nearest exam room and gently unrolled the soiled gauze and cotton bandaging around her feet. What we saw was enough to bring tears to our eyes. Her feet were swollen, red and horribly infected.

As we gently bathed her feet and brought her ibuprofen, antibiotics and water, we heard her story. Her older sister had been gang-raped in Central America because her brother had refused to join the local gang. This brave, young woman had escaped, walking across the desert in sneakers two sizes too small, starving and barely getting enough water until she found a ride to some relatives who lived near The Clinic.

The relatives reassured her that we would be compassionate and would treat her injuries without questions. And we did. We found her a spare winter coat, as it was now October, and we gave her shampoo and soap. We gave her our lunches. We gave her new bandaging, pain medicine and a huge hug. Her bravery touched every one of us at The Clinic.

In a time when so many live in fear, wondering if they're safe to go to the grocery store, to go to work or to visit the doctor, The Clinic is here to reassure them that our home is a safe place for them. We provide medical care without judgment. Medical care with love. Medical care without needless questions. That is medical care the The Clinic way.

Chapter Six: Addiction

The disease of addiction in our country has become an epidemic problem. The term addiction can be considered a generic term to include a number of disorders that include alcohol, cocaine, opiates, marijuana, gambling, Internet gaming, and overeating issues. Indeed, any activity that persistently interrupts a healthy life style might well be considered an addiction. Always fooling themselves, addicts always had a ready excuse for their behaviors, never knowing the doctors had actually heard all the excuses before. I submit a list, only partially tongue-in-cheek, of some of the more common.

How to lose a Percocet Prescription (or Explanations Given after a Failed Drug Test)

    1. I left it at the Shore/mountains/lake/on the

bus/at work/in my purse/in my car .

2. I put it on top of my car and it must have fallen off when I drove away.

3. It went through the wash.

4. I guess the pharmacy gave me the wrong number of pills.

5. My sister/aunt/ grandmother needed some, so I helped her out.

6. I had to spit one out and it dissolved in the sink before I could get it.

7. I thought you'd given me refills so I took it all.

8. Remember that flood? Well, my pills got washed right off my table and were lost! You remember that flood, don't you?

9. I was in a car accident, and the pill bottle got crushed....here it is....see????

10. My dog ate it.

Each of these is a real excuse, a real telephone call, a reason given for requesting more pain medicine.

Many of The Clinic's patients had real pain. Contractors with newly-herniated discs. Workers on their feet for 8 hours a day with acutely fractured metatarsals. Substitute teachers without medical benefits but with painful knee joints. People who HAD to work every day in order to feed their families.

People with no insurance, no opportunity to receive epidural back injections, no opportunity to obtain X-rays or physical therapy or steroid injections for their hip or knee arthritis: these people often needed a strong pain medication. And people, who unknowingly, with the brain chemistry pre-set by their DNA, became "high" on a narcotic instead of just having pain relief.

The Clinic certainly saw more unrelieved pain than a typical internal medicine or family practice office. For some, there was no choice but to "live with" the pain. And we certainly had to prescribe pain medication when a man with a herniated disc or hair-line fracture said, "Please, I HAVE to work, I have to get some groceries, or gas, or....."

There is a fine line between prescribing pain medications for those who truly need them and preventing others from acquiring them inappropriately. After a particularly bad two weeks when it seemed as if pain-medicine seekers were coming out of the woodwork, the staff and I retreated on a Friday after work, to a quiet corner in the local restaurant, to re-write our contract for controlled substances. Now, most medical practices which prescribe narcotic pain medicines have a "contract" which obliges the patient to follow certain guidelines, such as no early refills, no "lost" prescriptions and so on. Five or six of us sat with lined paper, some wine and good snacks, and created a two-page document which we felt would cover nearly all of the contingencies. The patient would have to read it aloud with a nurse and sign each item in the contract. And, indeed, it worked! Drug-seekers (without real pain) would be alarmed by the contingencies; those who used drugs recreationally would re-consider trying to obtain them at The Clinic. Those will real pain would happily sign the contract and co-operate with its guidelines.

Chapter Seven: Addiction treatment

In the USA at this time, there is an overwhelming abuse of opiates. Some patients are caught up in the narcotic cycle, started on pain medications by a specialist and then cut off. Others take narcotics for the high. For these patients we had a new approach.

At The Clinic, we recognized that opiate addiction was a mental health issue that was caused by a serious mood disorder and could be caused by a physical injury or a bout with depression, anxiety, poor self image, or anger issues.

It is vital to diagnose these mood problems and start the patient the proper medications as quickly as possible so that cognitive therapy can begin. In the case of opiates, a psychosocial approach is effective: appropriate medications, cognitive therapy, plus a positive approach to the patient can result in excellent results. With monitoring, weekly drug screens, and encouragement to attend recovery groups like NA and AA, patients have a good chance of managing and conquering their addictions.

At The Clinic, we tried to stem the mis-use of opioids very early on. We had an experienced Drug and Alcohol Counsellor whose resume includes at least a couple of decades at Bellevue Hospital in New York. We also had doctors who were conversant with the currently used meds for depression, bipolar disorder and anxiety, conditions which often led patients to mood-altering drugs and addiction.

We used Suboxone and Zubsolv with great success. These innovative drugs were office-based treatments for opiate addiction. Suboxone and Zubsolv were an opiate replacement, buprenorphine, with a blocker so that one would not become habituated or addicted to it and from which one could taper off. The use of this medication has dramatically curbed the urge to medicate oneself with opiate, and the use of this medicine meant no withdrawal symptoms from a medicine that could be handled in an office setting! This is distinctly different from methadone, highly addictive and not used in private practice.

Consider this: one woman, 62 years old with no history of any drug abuse or addiction, lost her job when she broke her hip after a fall. Sadly, she didn't break it at work, so it wasn't covered by Workers' Compensation insurance. She was treated by a charitably-minded orthopedist and hospital a few miles from our Clinic, but then found she couldn't stop taking her opiate pain medicine. Suboxone therapy worked, and over a course of a few months, she no longer needed the opiate (and the feelings of self-recrimination because of the addiction). She was able to receive sufficient Social Security Benefits to support her basic needs.

Our patients on buprenorphine therapy were "off the streets", no longer needed to buy drugs illegally, to steal, or to compromise themselves physically and morally. There is still much resistance in private practices to prescribing these drugs. "I don't want drug addicts in my office", "I don't know enough about it", "It's too time-consuming". But knowledge and proper use of these drugs , used by every physician, would certainly decrease the need to acquire opiates illegally and unsafely.

Chapter Eight: My Husband, Is He Having a Stroke?

On a lovely summer day in August, a frantic woman came in without an appointment. Her reluctant husband was with her.

"Look at his face," she said to the front desk volunteer. "It's lop-sided – I think he's having a stroke. He needs to see the doctor right now!"

The left side of his mouth did not move while the right side did, and his left eyelid drooped. He told us he could walk just fine and, no, he did not have a headache. His blood pressure was normal and the rest of his neurological exam was completely normal.

A stroke will usually affect a left eyelid and right side of the mouth, or vice versa, not one whole side of the face. There are two facial nerves, one on each side of the face. They control the movement of the muscles on that whole side. The drooping of the left eyelid and the left side of the mouth could only be due to paralysis of one facial nerve, not a problem in the brain itself.

Clearly, this was no stroke. This was Bell's Palsy, a paralysis (usually temporary) of the facial nerve.

In The Clinic's home of Chester County, Pennsylvania, Lyme disease is rampant. Indeed, the most common cause of Bell's Palsy in Pennsylvania (and much of the east coast of the United States) is Lyme disease. This infection will sometimes present with high fever, perhaps the typical "bulls-eye" rash and occasionally with a red, swollen and tender knee joint. At times, the symptoms are so minimal that they appear to be just a mild "summer flu." However, the Lyme bacteria is a sneaky sort of villain, a spirochete, and when the Lyme symptoms disappear, the spirochete does not always disappear with it.

Most bacterial infections, such as a streptococcal sore throat or a staphylococcus abscess, will respond to antibiotics and if they recur, it is probably a completely new infection. Even if the person has no access to antibiotics, there is a chance that the infections will resolve on their own, though in a much longer period of time. However, a spirochete such as Lyme goes through stages. In the first stage, there are symptoms of an acute infection, mild to severe. In the second stage, the spirochete is dormant, lying quietly, and there are no symptoms. The third stage is the vicious stage. The spirochete becomes active again and can cause damage to any system of the body, most particularly the neurological system. And this is what caused this man's Bell's Palsy.

If Bell's Palsy is treated quickly, with antibiotics directed toward the Lyme spirochete and prednisone for the inflammation of the nerve, most cases will resolve fairly quickly. But if there is no opportunity to see a doctor or to get treatment, the risk of permanent paralysis rises. a disability may develop, a disability which can be severe. The person may no longer be able to drink from a glass without spilling, and speech may be slurred because the lips do not move properly.

At The Clinic, we treated this man successfully, for the cost of a few antibiotic pills. His smile on recovery said it all.

Chapter Nine: How Do We Do It?

When we imagined The Clinic, one principle stood out: independence. We wanted to have a place for anyone to receive great medical care, and we did not want to be compelled to screen for income or birthplace or anything else not directly relevant to medical care.

This philosophy ruled out funding from a large number of possible supporting agencies, including the government, as so many agencies required much tighter guidelines that we cared to implement.

We have had, and continue to have, five major sources of funding for our ongoing work:

Each patient pays what he or she can afford to give. We have received a pocketful of loose change, we have received two crumpled dollar bills and we have received crisp $50 bills.

Private donations are of great importance in our keeping The Clinic thriving, covering the day-to-day expenses.   In the early years, we mailed out mimeographed typewritten letters to our donors, keeping them up-to-date on our patient flow and successes. Over time, we adopted professional-quality brochures and newsletters providing information and requests for donations. Some donors have given $10 a month every month since we opened; others send a quarterly check or a much-appreciated contribution at the end of the year. Our individual donors, along with our dedicated volunteers, are the lifeblood of The Clinic.

Foundations and corporate donors contribute about 60% of The Clinic's operating income. Although in our initial years we had to prove our stability to foundations in order to receive funding, over the years we have developed close relationships with several that fund us consistently every year. We also have a great appreciation for our corporate donors, who recognize the value of supporting the community where they work and live.

Church and community donors have also been very generous to The Clinic through the years. There are many philanthropy-minded towns across the US, but Phoenixville is a truly unique, special place when it comes to taking care of its neighbors.

Fundraisers have been an important way for The Clinic to both raise funds and connect with the community over the years. Since its inception, The Clinic has hosted an Annual Dinner, which eventually outgrew its smaller venue and expanded into a space that holds hundreds of guests. One year, we had a yard sale, spreading our wares all over the porch and lawn of The Clinic. Another year we held a book sale. Every little bit helps: one clever volunteer put out a five-gallon water jug, and volunteers and staff could drop in pocket change when they passed by. When that jug was filled, it would bring in some much-needed funds to restock supplies. For several years, The Clinic held a golf outing that was well-attended by individuals and businesses alike. Our newest fundraiser is an adult Field Day, in which teams compete in fun, quirky games to try to win the top prize. We are always looking for new ideas for events that our community will enjoy!

Along with our main sources of funding, we have many donors who make generous in-kind gifts. A few groups buy gifts and toys for our patients at the holidays. A local church delivers "flu bags" for our patients, filled with chicken soup, tea, throat lozenges, Tylenol and a thermometer. Winter coats, scarves and gloves are donated for the chilly months. We receive backpacks filled with supplies when it comes time for our youngest patients to go back to school, along with picture books, coloring books and crayons that they can enjoy at visits and then take home with them. One of our most generous partners is the Chester County Food Bank, which brings fresh fruit and vegetables for our patients every week, and even provided a refrigerator in which to store them.

Miracles happen too: one day when we realized we had no more postage stamps and no money to buy any. Half an hour later a passerby came in with a roll of 100 stamps. He told us he had been buying postage stamps at the post office and realized we might need some too. A divine intervention or miracle, for sure!

We receive donations ranging from very small to very large, and each and every one makes The Clinic's work possible.

Thank you to all these people and many, many more! The problem with starting to thank individuals is that very likely I will leave someone out.   If I do so, I humbly apologize.   Each and every volunteer made a difference to MY life and to the life of the patients at The Clinic.

Thank you especially to all the doctors who have volunteered:

Cardiology: Dr. Rajiv Dhawan and Dr. John Fornace

Dermatology: Dr. Dan Dvorkin and Linda Weinberg CRNP

Internal medicine/Family Practice: Dr. Steve Mark (who worked every week and made it possible for me to have an occasional afternoon off), Dr. Patty Boken, Dr. Ana Negron, Dr. Susan Prouty, Dr. Janet Brown, Dr Jeff Romeo, Dr. BettyAnne Hoepfner, Dr.Dana Greenblatt, Anne Haney, CRNP

Gynecology: Dr. Jim Kolter, Dr. Nancy Hahn, Dr. Allyson Brown, Dr. Amy Jane Cadieux, Rosalie Lisa, CRNP

Urology: Dr. Gus Spector, Dr. Thomas Lanchoney, Dr. Peter Oskanian

Allergy: Dr. Sumita Roy-Ghanta

Ophthalmology: Dr. Dan Kane

Pediatrics: Dr. Ned Keinzle (who has worked since the opening of The Clinic in 2002, undoubtedly the longest-serving volunteer). I also thank him for being an excellent source of trivia questions; Dr Jeff Bomze

Orthopedics: Dr Glenn Lipton, Dr. Guille

Plastic and hand surgery: Dr Frank DeLone

Psychology: Dr. Jane Buhl, Katie Hynes

Psychiatry: Dr. Faith Midwood, Dr. Al Derivan, Dr. Doeff

Therapists: Ed Barrett, Cara Graver, Jody Dill, Betsy Bouvel

Paramedic : Jesse Kontra

HUGE thanks to our Boards of Directors!

The Reverend Marie Swayze helped make The Clinic happen. The Clinic owes her a huge debt of gratitude. To her late husband, Richard, too, a man who could fix "anything" and frequently did just that for us, including on a Sunday morning, when a flood from the burst hot water heater on the third floor spilled into the second and then the first floor, making EVERYTHING wet.   MaryEllen Smith was my right-hand-person in the lab, in the med room and with publicity. Anne Reid has been a part of The Clinic, from its earliest imagination to being a long time volunteer then Office Manager and Volunteer Co-ordinator.   Dr. Susan Prouty worked 3 days a week as an internist since nearly the opening of The Clinic, and she was a constant pleasure to work with, to consult with, and to plan with. Could never have had a vacation if she hadn't been there. And her handwriting was legible!

Our volunteer nurses, medical assistants, students, clerical workers, translators, THANK YOU!   Our

Church partners, THANK YOU! Our foundations, THANK YOU!   To Paoli Hospital, who made it possibfor our patients to obtain radiology studies, THANK YOU! To our individual donors, THANK YOU. And to Beth Flor, Director of Development at The Clinic, for editing these pages, THANK YOU.

You have made a difference in the world.